Yoga

**An Introductory to Yoga for mind,
Body and Spirit**

Kim Fyffe

This book is dedicated to anyone looking to achieve inner peace, mental clarity and focus, flexibility, weight loss, and improved health from the practice of yoga.

Copyright Act of 1976, the scanning, uploading and electronic sharing of any part of this book without the explicit written consent or permission of the publisher constitutes unlawful piracy and the theft of intellectual property.

If you would like to use material or content from this book (other than for review purposes), prior written permission must be obtained from the publisher.

You can contact the publishing company at admin@speedypublishing.com. Thank you for not infringing on the author's rights.

Speedy Publishing LLC (c) 2014
40 E. Main St., #1156
Newark, DE 19711
www.speedypublishing.co

Ordering Information:
Quantity sales; Special discounts are available on quantity purchases by corporations, associations, and others. For details, contact the "Special Sales Department" at the address above.

This is a reprint book.

Manufactured in the United States of America

TABLE OF CONTENTS

Publisher's Notes i

Chapter 1: Introduction to Yoga 1

Chapter 2: The Benefits of Yoga 5

Chapter 3: Tips for Anyone New To Yoga 10

Chapter 4: Yoga Equipment – Do You Need It? 12

Chapter 5: The Different Types of Yoga 17

Chapter 6: 12 Yoga Poses to Get You Started 22

Chapter 7: What Is Meditation? 43

Chapter 8: Yoga at Your Desk 52

Chapter 9: Yoga Poses to Relieve Headaches, Cramps and Depression 55

Chapter 10: Conclusion 67

Meet the Author 69

Publisher's Notes

Disclaimer

This publication is intended to provide helpful and informative material. It is not intended to diagnose, treat, cure, or prevent any health problem or condition, nor is intended to replace the advice of a physician. No action should be taken solely on the contents of this book. Always consult your physician or qualified health-care professional on any matters regarding your health and before adopting any suggestions in this book or drawing inferences from it.

The author and publisher specifically disclaim all responsibility for any liability, loss or risk, personal or otherwise, which is incurred as a consequence, directly or indirectly, from the use or application of any contents of this book.

Any and all product names referenced within this book are the trademarks of their respective owners. None of these owners have sponsored, authorized, endorsed, or approved this book.

Always read all information provided by the manufacturers' product labels before using their products. The author and publisher are not responsible for claims made by manufacturers.

Chapter 1: Introduction to Yoga

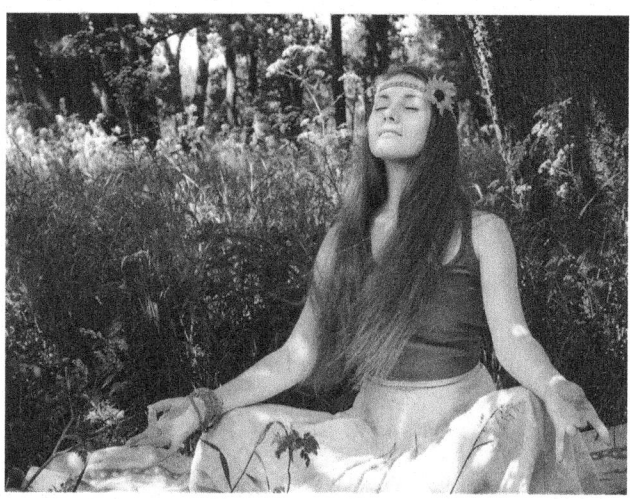

What Is Yoga?

When one mentions "yoga", many images may be conjured up. Perhaps you get an image of flower children from the 60's sitting in a circle with their legs in impossible positions chanting "Ohm" around a huge candle in a poorly lit room. Yoga is an ancient art that has been practiced for centuries. Over the years, it has risen in popularity as a way to stay fit, get in touch with one's inner self, and keep a balance of sanity in a sometimes insane world.

While yoga did come to popularity in the 60's with Maharishi Mahesh Yogi who popularized Transcendental Meditation (TM) in the 60's, because he was associated with the Beatles, yoga practitioners have brought the ancient practice to the forefront of wellness in recent years.

Many scholars believe that yoga dates back over 5,000 years to the beginning of human civilization. Scholars believe that yoga grew out of Stone Age Shamanism, because of the cultural similarities between Modern Hinduism and Mehrgarh, a neolithic settlement (in what is now Afghanistan). In fact, much of Hindu ideas, rituals and symbols of today appear to have their roots in this shamanistic culture of Mehrgarh.

Early Yoga and archaic shamanism had much in common as both sought to transcend the human condition. The primary goal of shamanism was to heal members of the community and act as religious mediators. Archaic Yoga was also community oriented, as it attempted to discern the cosmic order through inner vision, then to apply that order to daily living. Later, Yoga evolved into a more inward experience, and Yogis focused on their individual enlightenment and salvation.

Yoga is the most diversified spiritual practice in the world. Crossing over many cultures (including Hinduism, Buddhism, Jainism and the West), Yoga also extends over multiple languages such as Hindi, Tibetan, Bengali, Sanskrit, Tamil, Prakit, Marathi and Pali. The Yogic tradition continues to proliferate and spread its message of peace to this very day.

There are many different places that offer yoga classes – gyms, wellness centers, even the local YMCA. But you don't have to join a class to practice yoga. It is just as easily done in your home or even at your desk while at work. Yoga can help bring you inner peace when you are stressed out. It can even help relieve the pain of headaches, backaches, and menstrual cramps.

As studies continue to reveal yoga's many health benefits, this centuries-old Eastern philosophy is fast becoming the new fitness soul mate for workout enthusiasts. Contemporary devotees range from high-powered execs trying to keep hearts beating on a healthy note to image-conscious Hollywood stars striving for sleek physiques. Even prominent athletes are adding yoga to their training regime to develop balanced, injury-free muscles and spines.

Yet to applaud yoga for its physical benefits alone would only diminish what this entire system has to offer as a whole. By practicing yoga on a regular basis, you may be surprised to find that you're building much more than a strong, flexible body.

Initially, the sole purpose of practicing yoga was to experience spiritual enlightenment. In Sanskrit (the ancient language of India), yoga translates as "yoke" or "union," describing the integration of mind and body to create a greater connection with one's own pure, essential nature.

Classes that have gained popularity in the United States usually teach one of the many types of hatha yoga, a physical discipline which focuses mainly on asanas (postures) and breath work in order to prepare the body for spiritual pursuits.

We will attempt to simplify the ancient practice of yoga by showing you some basic yoga positions, giving you tips on performing yoga exercises, and inducting meditation practices into your everyday life. Through yoga and meditation, you could come to a new level of enlightenment with your personal life and enhance the quality of your existence.

No longer is yoga a mysterious phenomenon. It is now simply a way to keep you healthy and aligned. Now relax and read on as we explore yoga and meditation.

Misconceptions about Yoga

Yoga is far more than just a series of stretching exercises. It's not some kind of religion or cult, and it doesn't require one to turn into a vegan or sell all of their worldly possessions! It's nothing like its stereotype.

Yoga first came to the Western hemisphere in 1893 at the World's Fair in Chicago. It was brought by Swami Vivekananda who was one of India's most popular gurus.

The word yoga gets its origins from the Sanskrit word "Yug". It means to bind or join. Basically it is about unity of the physical body with the mind. It's about "conscious living".

It's not all about calisthenics. While the physical aspects are certainly an important part, this is not the only true purpose. It's also about the mental benefits.

It's not any type of religion. There are no gods to worship, and it is not an organized system at all. Any spiritual benefits are purely emotional and psychological.

Yoga doesn't actually distinguish between the physical body and the mind. Yoga can work to improve your physical health in many ways, not just aiding in weight loss, but also improving tone and even reducing physical pain.

Yoga allows you to release the tension that can build up in your body. It helps the various parts of your body become lose and limber, from your muscles and joints to your tendons and ligaments. It can help back pain, joint pain, muscle pain, and much more.

People aren't meant to be stiff and rigid. We were designed to be flexible creatures. We may not all have the flexibility and grace of a prima ballerina, but we should all be healthy and fit. Yoga is one means to achieving such a goal.

Chapter 2: The Benefits of Yoga

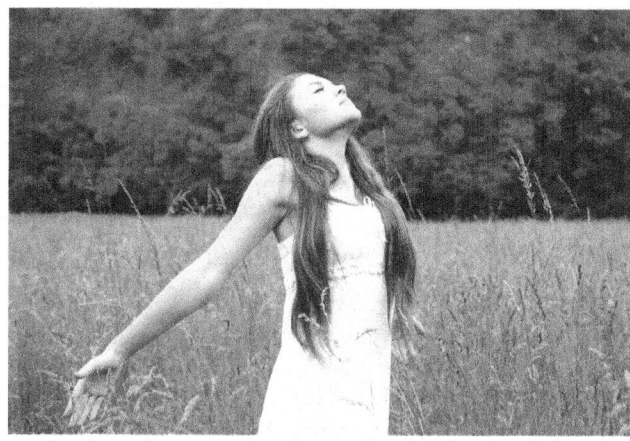

Yoga Creates both flexibility and strength along with cardiovascular health. It creates mental clarity and focus and emotional balance. Yoga is safe for all ages and body types. It facilitates healing from injuries and is a wonderful way to create wellness.

You weight train to gain strength, jog or do aerobics for a cardiovascular workout, practice tai-chi to develop a sense of balance and harmony, stretch to gain flexibility, and meditate to develop peace of mind and relaxation. Yoga is a form of exercise that gives you everything: strength, endurance, balance, flexibility, and relaxation. It is the only complete form of bodywork that does it all. Indeed, yoga is more than stretching and relaxation: it is the ultimate mind-body challenge.

Yoga increases flexibility as it offers positions that act upon the various joints of the body including those joints that aren't always in the forefront of noticeability. These joints are rarely exercised, however, with yoga, they are!

Various yoga positions exercise the different tendons and ligaments of the body. The body that may have been quite rigid begins experiencing a remarkable flexibility in even those parts which have not been consciously worked upon. Seemingly unrelated non-strenuous yoga positions act upon certain parts of the body in an interrelated manner. When done together, they work in harmony to create a situation where flexibility is attained relatively easily.

Yoga is perhaps the only form of activity which massages all the internal glands and organs of the body in a thorough manner, including those – such as the prostate - that hardly get externally stimulated during our entire lifetime. Yoga acts in a wholesome manner on the various body parts. This stimulation and massage of the organs in turn benefits us by keeping away disease and providing a forewarning at the first possible instance of a likely onset of disease or disorder.

By gently stretching muscles and joints as well as massaging the various organs, yoga ensures the optimum blood supply to various parts of the body. This helps in the flushing out of toxins from every nook and cranny as well as providing nourishment up to the last point. This leads to benefits such as delayed ageing, energy and a remarkable zest for life.

But these enormous physical benefits are just a "side effect" of this powerful practice. What yoga does is harmonize the mind with the body. This results in real quantum benefits. It is now an open secret that the will of the mind has enabled people to achieve extraordinary physical feats, which proves beyond doubt the mind and body connection.

Yoga through meditation works remarkably to achieve this harmony and helps the mind work in sync with the body. How often do we find that we are unable to perform our activities properly and in a satisfying manner because of the confusions and conflicts in our mind weigh down heavily upon us? Moreover, stress which in reality is the #1 killer affecting all parts of our physical, endocrinal and emotional systems can be corrected through the wonderful yoga practice of meditation.

In fact yoga = meditation, because both work together in achieving the common goal of unity of mind, body and spirit – a state of eternal bliss.

The meditative practices through yoga help in achieving an emotional balance through detachment. What it means is that meditation creates conditions, where you are not affected by the happenings around you. This in turn creates a remarkable calmness and a positive outlook, which also has tremendous benefits on the physical health of the body.

There's no doubt that yoga has tremendous benefits to your health and well-being. So how do you get started with your own yoga program? Let's look at the basic styles of yoga and what they mean.

Benefits That Have Been Proven To Exist Through Yoga

- ✓ Improved flexibility
- ✓ Better range of motion
- ✓ More fluid motion
- ✓ Immune system strengthening
- ✓ Reduced joint pain
- ✓ Reduced muscular pain
- ✓ Better breathing
- ✓ Higher lung capacity
- ✓ Higher metabolism
- ✓ Better sleep quality
- ✓ Reduced stress and anxiety

There are many other remarkable benefits reported to be received from yoga. You may discover many more.

Yoga is beneficial in many ways. It's not all about the physical effects, as I've mentioned previously. Yoga may have its roots in the spiritual, but its foundation is based in science.

Yoga's health benefits have been proven time and time again by many sources. Its physical benefits can be paramount to a healthy lifestyle.

But of course there are mental and emotional benefits, as well. Yoga helps you achieve a type of mind/body harmony through the use of:

- ✓ Postures (called asana)
- ✓ Breathing (called pranayama)
- ✓ Meditation (which we will cover later)

All three of these are essential for obtaining the full benefit of yoga. For example, you may believe your breathing has nothing to do with your physical shape, but that's not true. Your body needs oxygen to function properly, and the more efficient your respiration is, the better your body can perform.

Likewise meditation can also help you physically. When you meditate you relieve muscle tension. This can ease all kinds of aches and pains including back pain, joint pain, and even stress and anxiety.

There are a number of direct physical benefits that can be obtained from yoga when you use the three principles together:

- ✓ Central nervous system harmony
- ✓ Decrease in heart rate
- ✓ Lower blood pressure
- ✓ Better efficiency of your cardiovascular system
- ✓ Gastrointestinal system improvement
- ✓ Improved flexibility and dexterity
- ✓ Better balance
- ✓ Better memory and mental clarity
- ✓ Depth perception improvement

There are a number of psychological benefits, too:

- ✓ Can help break a smoking habit
- ✓ Can help curb binge drinking
- ✓ Can help you eat healthier

- ✓ Can help ease insomnia
- ✓ Can reduce stress and anxiety
- ✓ Can decrease panic attacks
- ✓ Can ease depression
- ✓ Can help lethargy

While yoga isn't a cure-all and results won't happen overnight, it can certainly help you make some big changes to your psychological and physiological states.

There are even some claims out there that yoga can ease the symptoms of many other illnesses, like diabetes. This has never been proven by medical science, but some people claim it can reduce the need for insulin by up to 50%.

Yoga is also something that is relatively easy on the body. You can tailor a yoga workout to your own fitness level, and increase the difficulty as you progress.

There's no reason you shouldn't be able to perform at least some of the asana no matter what physical condition you're in. As long as you have some mobility in your arms and legs, you should be able to start out with some of the easier asana and gradually increase the intensity of your yoga workout as you progress.

Don't overdo it. Too much of a good thing can be bad for you. You want to use yoga to improve your physical condition, not make it worse.

If you overdo it, you may end up injuring yourself. This could make existing conditions worse and also set back any progress you've made so far.

At the very least an injury could cause you to miss several days of workouts, which could hamper your progress, so it's best to take it easy until you get used to it.

Chapter 3: Tips for Anyone New To Yoga

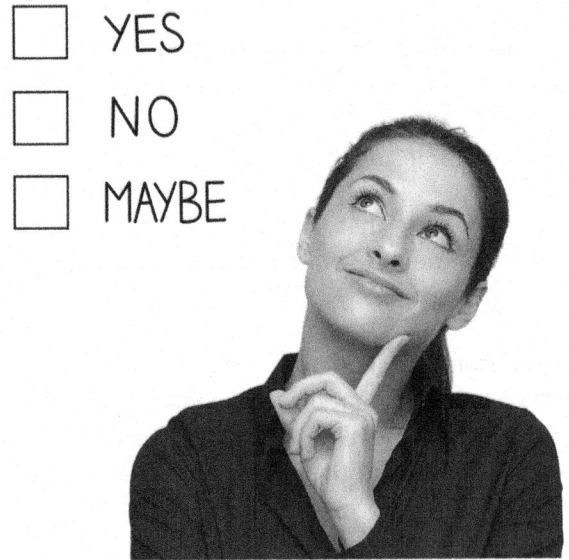

Yoga has been proven to have many different health benefits, both psychological and physiological. It is an ancient practice, but it has very practical applications in this new day and age.

Before you get started with yoga you might want to ask yourself a few questions. These are meant to get your mind into the right mindset before you begin.

- Why do I want to start yoga?
- Are my goals realistic?
- Do I have any physical limitations that might put me at greater risk of injury than other people?

- Do I have clear and definable goals?
- Am I ready to commit to a program?
- Will my family and friends support me, and if they don't, will I be able to handle it?

When looking for a yoga instructor, you might want to visit a few of their classes first to get a feel for the style of the individual. Some people claim to be yoga instructors but actually know very little about it. So that is an obvious concern.

You may also have to deal with instructors who are angry or violent. This is unusual, but it has been known to happen. Some instructors are very "innovative", and I say that carefully because this isn't always a good thing.

A few rare instructors have been known to run their classes more like a boot camp than a yoga class. They deviate from the true path of yoga in order to chase the almighty dollar by doing something "unique". But you can't get into the true spirit of yoga if you're being yelled at, degraded, and stressed out!

Yoga is about calmness, peace, and tranquility. It is also about discipline, yes, but not in a drill sergeant kind of way! The discipline comes from careful control of the mind and body by the individual, not by an outside source.

If your yoga classes end up making you feel uncomfortable or upset, then you must question their value to you. When a class causes more stress than it eliminates, you should seriously rethink your choice to join it.

Look for a class that looks fun and an instructor you like and feel comfortable with. The more at ease you are in the class, the more successful it will be for you.

Chapter 4: Yoga Equipment – Do You Need It?

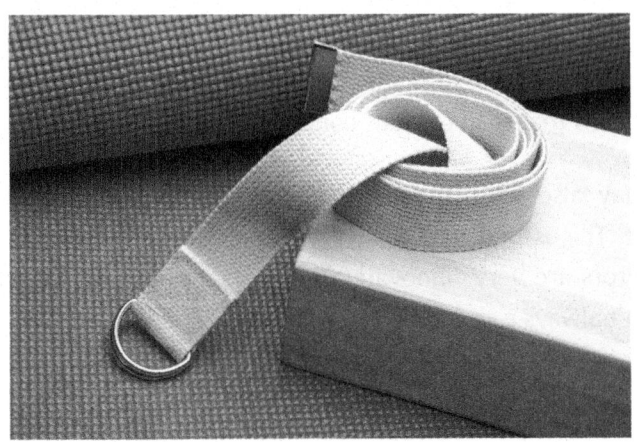

There are many items available for those who practice yoga. None of them are truly required, but there are many that would be especially helpful.

You may have even seen a number of them in videos, on television, or in your local store. Perhaps you didn't even realize they were used for yoga.

For many years yoga equipment was hard to find and somewhat expensive. Now it's very prevalent and the prices on most equipment are very affordable.

The problem is, the prevalence of equipment makes it hard to decide what you need and what you don't. You don't need everything, no matter what the salesperson may try to tell you.

We're going to look at some of the most popular types of yoga equipment and accessories so you can decide what you need, what you might want, and what you can live without.

If you're just getting started you really need very little, especially if you'll be taking a class. Your class may provide the items you need, but not all will. You'll probably need to bring your own mat at the very least.

The equipment you buy will also largely be a personal choice. You may not need to buy something that someone else would consider essential.

For example, you'll find some people who prefer to sit on a hard floor or on the ground outdoors. Others find it very uncomfortable to sit on a hard surface and may feel pain in their back and tailbone. These people would really need a yoga mat.

I'm going to simply describe each item and let you make your own judgments as to what is right for you. I won't try to tell you what you should and shouldn't buy, but I will tell you what I feel might be helpful.

Yoga Mats

For most people, a yoga mat will be essential. A lot of people won't be able to comfortably sit on the floor without a mat, and this can be very discouraging. You may be fine without one, but it's something you should consider.

The first thing you should look for in a yoga mat is a good floor grip. You're not going to want a mat that will slip around a lot, especially while you're attempting difficult postures.

You'll also want to choose a mat with enough padding to make it comfortable.

You'll find yoga mats in different sizes, thicknesses, and colors, so you'll be able to find one to suit you. If you're going to buy one, you should be sure to find one that you're really happy with.

Yoga Towel

There are special towels that are made for yoga. You may find super-absorbent towels that will be quite helpful if you sweat a lot, and you may even find these in "chakra colors" which you can use in various situations.

You may also buy a skidless towel that you can use on your mat to help absorb sweat. This may be especially important if you practice Bikram yoga.

Yoga Bags

If you buy a lot of yoga accessories you may want to buy a special bag to carry them. They look like duffel bags, and are often made of nylon.

You can find these bags in many stores, and they range from around $10 up to $50 or $100.

Yoga Straps

If you have trouble holding your poses you might wish to buy yoga straps. They can help you hold those difficult poses longer.

Yoga Sandbags and Bolsters

Sandbags and bolsters can help you keep your balance and support you through your poses. They come in many colors, and you may be able to match your outfit, mat, and other accessories.

Yoga Meditation Seating

Meditation seating comes in a variety of different types. You can buy special cushions, benches, and pillows for various poses, and they make it very comfortable for meditating for longer periods of time.

Yoga Balls

For around $25 you can buy a yoga ball. They help you learn balance, build your strength, tone your muscles, and make it comfortable for people with injuries to exercise.

These balls provide extra support as you stretch, and are good for working out the back and hips, and can also be used during pregnancy.

You'll need an air pump if you get one of these. The air will slowly come out of the ball as you use it, causing it to deflate after several uses, so you shouldn't forget to buy a pump to fill it back up.

Yoga Blocks

Yoga blocks are somewhat like mattresses. They have a number of uses, but they are most commonly used for body movement extensions.

Yoga Videos

Many people love to pick up videos they can use at home. They may not have the money for formal classes, or they may feel shy or awkward about attending classes with other people. Perhaps they just don't have a lot of extra time.

Videos are a really good way to get into yoga if you can't take formal yoga classes. You'll be able to get in more practice and feel more comfortable doing some of the poses at home. If you decide later to take formal classes you'll already be a little ahead of some of the others in the class, especially if you start in beginners' classes.

Yoga Music

There are special CDs you can buy that are made to enhance the meditation experience. These can be used for enhancing the tranquility you experience.

There are also CDs that help with your flow, including trance music. You may also find chants and mantras on CD that can help you get into the right frame of mind.

Yoga Clothing

You don't need any special clothing for practicing yoga unless you just want to buy some. Many people like to exercise in full leotards of different types, but a comfortable cotton t-shirt and stretchy leggings that breathe would be just fine.

Chapter 5: The Different Types of Yoga

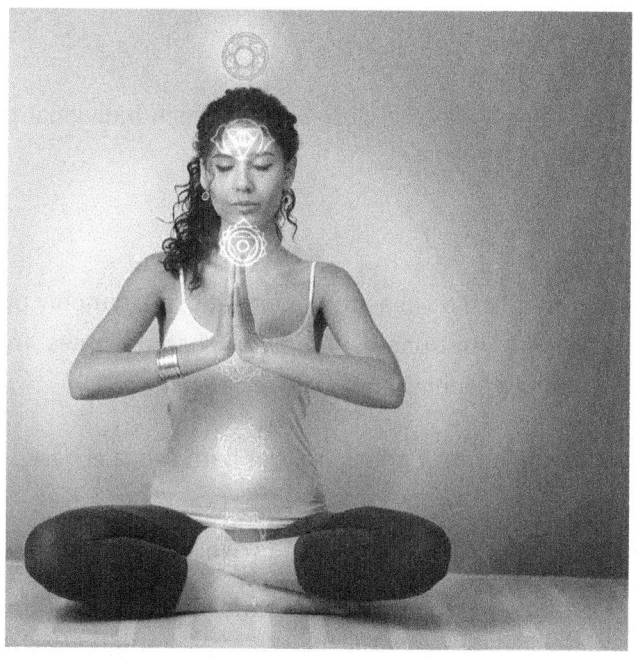

There are several different types of yoga. Most people just think of yoga as being one standard set of poses, but it's not quite that simple.

Western yoga is generally just defined as "yoga". There aren't usually any types mentioned. Western yoga often uses a mixture of different yoga types, and different instructors may even come up with their own poses or mix their own unique blends.

There are in fact six types of yoga traditionally practiced, plus a new type, bikram yoga, that has been rapidly gaining in popularity recently.

The six traditional types of yoga are:

1. Hatha
2. Raja
3. Karma
4. Bhakti
5. Jnana
6. Tantra

Now we're going to take a closer look at each individual types of yoga and their differences.

Hatha Yoga

The teachings of hatha yoga are the type most commonly practiced in the Western hemisphere. The word hatha comes from the Sanskrit term ha (meaning sun).

There are two important principles that hatha yoga is based on:

1. **Meditation** – You will find at least one posture that is especially comfortable to you and that you can sustain for long period of time while you meditate. As you advance, you'll ideally learn several postures that you are comfortable with. Many people find the lotus position especially helpful for meditation.
2. **Improving Energy Within The Body** – This is all about improving the flow of energy throughout your body so improve your overall health.

Raja Yoga

Raja yoga is also known as "classical yoga" very similar to hatha yoga. Raja is considered a bit more difficult than other forms of yoga, because it requires more discipline and control than other forms.

Raja yoga focuses on concentration, meditation, and discipline of the mind and body.

There are eight limbs of raja yoga:

1. *Yama* – Ethical standards
2. *Niyama* - Self discipline - Self restraint
3. *Asana* - Posture
4. *Pranayama* - Breath control
5. *Pratyahara* – Sensory withdrawl
6. *Dharana* - Concentration
7. *Dhyana* - Meditation
8. *Samadhi* - Ecstasy (not the drug!)

Karma Yoga

The word karma means "action". Karma is generally thought of as the unseen force in the world that causes good things to happen to good people and bad things to pay back those who have done wrong.

Karma yoga means selfless action. To perform karma yoga, you are supposed to surrender yourself completely to serve the greater good - the good of man and humanity.

The founder of karma yoga is Bhagavad Vita. This version is heavily rooted in Hinduism. Although you don't have to practice Hinduism to practice karma yoga, you should potentially familiarize yourself with the teachings of Hinduism in order to fully understand and appreciate karma yoga.

Bhakti Yoga

Bhatki yoga is a sensual, erotic form of yoga. It's all about love, divine love, specifically.

Love operates on three levels according the principles of bhatki yoga:

1. Material love
2. Human love
3. Spiritual love

Jnana Yoga

Jnana yoga is all about wisdom and enlightenment. It's about clearing the mind and the soul and releasing negativity. It's about transformation and taking the path to true enlightenment.

Tantra Yoga

Tantra yoga is perhaps the type of yoga people are most curious about. It's not about sex exclusively, but that is a part of it. It is about reaching enlightenment and transcending the self through several rituals.

Sex is indeed one of those rituals, but it is not the only one by any means. Some tantric practitioners even recommend a life of celibacy.

Tantra means "expansion". The aim of tantra yoga is to expand your mind so that you can reach all levels of consciousness. It uses rituals to bring out the male and female aspects within an individual in order to awake the true spirit within.

Bikram Yoga

Bikram yoga is a relatively new form of yoga. It is not included in the six traditional forms of yoga, but it is becoming so popular it deserves a very special mention.

Bikram yoga was developed by Bikram Choudhury. It takes place in a room that is at 105°F with a humidity of about 40%. There are 26 postures and two types of breathing exercises.

Bikram yoga is more about detoxifying the body rather than reaching some sort of spiritual enlightenment. By forcing the body to sweat profusely, toxins are eliminated through the skin.

Additionally, the extra warmth makes the body more flexible, which helps prevent injury, relieves stress, and helps aid in deeper stretching.

Some people oppose Bikram yoga because it defeats the very principles of yoga. It has been heavily commercialized, and its creators protect it by copyright.

CHAPTER 6: 12 YOGA POSES TO GET YOU STARTED

Yoga is less workout and more mind-body exploration. Workout implies sweating as you push your body into exercise mode. That isn't what yoga is about.

So, here's a good way to start your yoga plan. Do these exercises in the order given for a good beginning workout.

Easy Pose

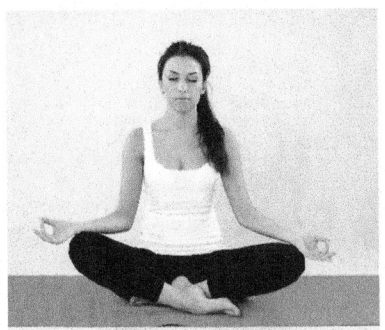

Begin with the easy pose. Easy pose is a comfortable seated position for meditation. This pose opens the hips, lengthens the spine and promotes grounding and inner calm. Basically, you're sitting cross legged like you did in school as a young child. "Criss cross apple sauce", as my teacher used to say!

With the buttocks on the floor, cross your legs and place your feet directly below your knees. Rest your hands on your knees with the palms facing up.

Press your hip bones down into the floor and reach the crown of the head up to lengthen the spine. Drop your shoulders down and back and press your chest towards the front of the room.

Relax your face, jaw, and belly. Let your tongue rest on the roof of your mouth just behind your front teeth. Breathe deeply through the nose down into the belly and hold as long as is comfortable.

<u>Downward-Facing Dog</u>

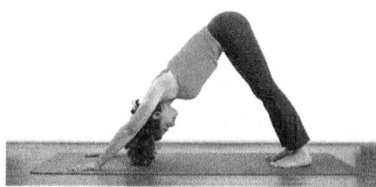

After the easy pose, move into downward-facing dog. This is one of the most widely recognized yoga poses. Downward-Facing Dog is an all-over, rejuvenating stretch.

Benefits include:

- Calms the brain and helps relieve stress and mild depression
- Energizes the body
- Stretches the shoulders, hamstrings, calves, arches, and hands
- Strengthens the arms and legs
- Helps relieve the symptoms of menopause
- Relieves menstrual discomfort when done with head supported
- Helps prevent osteoporosis
- Improves digestion
- Relieves headache, insomnia, back pain, and fatigue

- Therapeutic for high blood pressure, asthma, flat feet, sciatica, sinusitis

Use caution doing this pose if you have carpal tunnel syndrome, are in the late stages of pregnancy, or suffer from high blood pressure.

Come onto the floor on your hands and knees. Set your knees directly below your hips and your hands slightly forward of your shoulders. Spread your palms, index fingers parallel or slightly turned out, and turn your toes under.

Exhale and lift your knees away from the floor. At first keep the knees slightly bent and the heels lifted away from the floor. Lengthen your tailbone away from the back of your pelvis and press it lightly toward the pubis. Against this resistance, lift the sitting bones toward the ceiling, and from your inner ankles draw the inner legs up into the groins.

Then with an exhalation, push your top thighs back and stretch your heels onto or down toward the floor. Straighten your knees but be sure not to lock them. Firm the outer thighs and roll the upper thighs inward slightly. Narrow the front of the pelvis.

Firm the outer arms and press the bases of the index fingers actively into the floor. From these two points, lift along your inner arms from the wrists to the tops of the shoulders. Firm your shoulder blades against your back then widen them and draw them toward the tailbone. Keep the head between the upper arms; don't let it hang.

Stay in this pose anywhere from 1 to 3 minutes. Then bend your knees to the floor with an exhalation and rest.

Sun Salutations

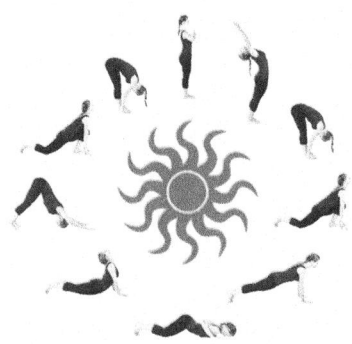

On days when you think you have no time for yoga, try and do at least one or two rounds of the Sun Salutation. You'll feel the difference.

After downward-facing dog, move into 3 rounds of sun salutations.

Stand facing the direction of the sun with both feet touching. Bring the hands together, palm-to-palm, at the heart. Inhale and raise the arms upward. Slowly bend backward, stretching arms above the head. Exhale slowly bending forward, touching the earth with respect until the hands are in line with the feet, head touching knees.

Inhale and move the right leg back away from the body in a wide backward step. Keep the hands and feet firmly on the ground, with the left foot between the hands. Raise the head. While exhaling, bring the left foot together with the right.

Keep arms straight, raise the hips and align the head with the arms, forming an upward arch. Exhale and lower the body to the floor until the feet, knees, hands, chest, and forehead are touching the ground. Inhale and slowly raise the head and bend backward as much as possible, bending the spine to the maximum.

While exhaling, bring the left foot together with the right. Keep arms straight, raise the hips and align the head with the arms, forming an upward arch. Inhale and move the right leg back away from the body in a wide backward step.

Keep the hands and feet firmly on the ground, with the left foot between the hands. Raise the head. Exhale slowly bending forward, touching the earth with respect until the hands are in line with the feet, head touching knees.

Inhale and raise the arms upward. Slowly bend backward, stretching arms above the head. Stand facing the direction of the sun with both feet touching. Bring the hands together, palm-to-palm, at the heart.

Tree Pose - Vriksha Asana

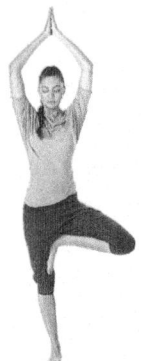

Benefits include:

- Strengthens thighs, calves, ankles, and spine
- Stretches the groins and inner thighs, chest and shoulders
- Improves sense of balance
- Relieves sciatica and reduces flat feet

Use caution if you suffer from insomnia or low blood pressure. If you have high blood pressure, do not raise your arms above your head.

Stand with the feet together and the arms by your sides. Bend the right leg at the knee, raise the right thigh and bring the sole of the right foot as high up the inside of the left thigh as possible.

Balancing on the left foot, raise both arms over the head, keep the elbows unbent and join the palms together. Hold the posture while breathing gently through the nostrils for about 10 complete breaths.

Lower the arms and right leg and return to the tad-asana, standing position with feet together and arms at the sides. Pause for a few moments and repeat on the opposite leg. Do this two or three times per leg or as long as is comfortable.

The challenge of the *vriksha-asana* is maintaining balance on one leg. Poor balance is often the result of a restless mind or distracted attention. Regular practice of this posture will help focus the mind and cultivate concentration (*dharana*).

When practicing *vriksha-asana* it may help to imagine or picture a tree in the mind and apply the following technique: Imagine that the foot you are balanced on is the root of the tree and the leg is the trunk.

Continue by imagining the head and outstretched arms as the branches and leaves of the tree. You may be unsteady for a while and find the body swaying back and forth, but don't break the concentration. Like a tree bending in the wind and yet remaining upright, the body can maintain balance.

Aim to achieve the "rootedness" and firmness of a tree. Regular practice of the *vriksha-asana* improves concentration, balance and coordination. Because the weight of the entire body is balanced on one foot, the muscles of that leg are strengthened and toned as well.

As you advance in this posture and are able to remain standing for more than a few moments, try closing the eyes and maintaining your balance.

Extended Triangle Pose

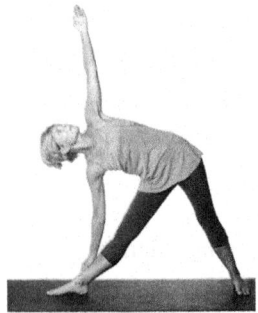

Benefits include:

- Stretches and strengthens the thighs, knees, and ankles
- Stretches the hips, groins, hamstrings, and calves; shoulders, chest, and spine
- Stimulates the abdominal organs
- Helps relieve stress
- Improves digestion
- Helps relieve the symptoms of menopause
- Relieves backache, especially through second trimester of pregnancy
- Therapeutic for anxiety, flat feet, infertility, neck pain, osteoporosis, and sciatica.

Use caution if you suffer from low blood pressure, have a heart condition, or have neck problems.

Stand with the feet together and the arms by your sides. Separate the feet slightly further than shoulder distance apart. Inhale and raise both arms straight out from the shoulders parallel to the floor with the palms facing down.

Exhale slowly while turning the torso to the left, bend at the waist and bring the right hand down to the left ankle. The palm of the right hand is placed along the outside of the left ankle. The left arm should be extended upward. Both legs and arms are kept straight without bending the knees and elbows.

Turn the head upward to the left and gaze up at the fingertips of the left hand. Inhale and return to a standing position with the arms outstretched. Hold this position for the duration of the exhaled breath. Exhale and repeat on the opposite side.

The triangle pose is basically doing slow toe touches while concentrating on your breathing and stretching your body.

Seated Forward Bend – Paschimottanasana

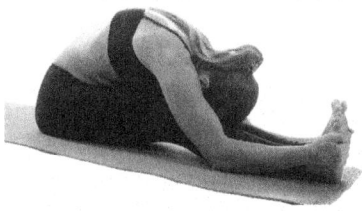

Literally translated as "intense stretch of the west," Paschimottanasana can help a distracted mind unwind.

Benefits include:

- Calms the brain and helps relieve stress and mild depression

- Stretches the spine, shoulders, hamstrings
- Stimulates the liver, kidneys, ovaries, and uterus
- Improves digestion
- Helps relieve the symptoms of menopause and menstrual discomfort
- Soothes headache and anxiety and reduces fatigue
- Therapeutic for high blood pressure, infertility, insomnia, and sinusitis
- Traditional texts say that Paschimottanasana increases appetite, reduces obesity, and cures diseases

Use caution if you suffer from asthma or have a back injury.

Sit on the floor with your buttocks supported on a folded blanket and your legs straight in front of you. Press actively through your heels. Rock slightly onto your left buttock, and pull your right sitting bone away from the heel with your right hand. Repeat on the other side.

Turn the top thighs in slightly and press them down into the floor. Press through your palms or finger tips on the floor beside your hips and lift the top of the sternum toward the ceiling as the top thighs descend.

Draw the inner groins deep into the pelvis. Inhale, and keeping the front torso long, lean forward from the hip joints, not the waist. Lengthen the tailbone away from the back of your pelvis. If possible take the sides of the feet with your hands, thumbs on the soles, elbows fully extended; if this isn't possible, loop a strap around the foot soles, and hold the strap firmly. Be sure your elbows are straight, not bent.

When you are ready to go further, don't forcefully pull yourself into the forward bend, whether your hands are on the feet or holding the strap. Always lengthen the front torso into the pose, keeping your head raised.

If you are holding the feet, bend the elbows out to the sides and lift them away from the floor; if holding the strap, lighten your grip and walk the hands forward, keeping the arms long. The lower belly should touch the thighs first, then the upper belly, then the ribs, and the head last.

With each inhalation, lift and lengthen the front torso just slightly; with each exhalation release a little more fully into the forward bend. In this way the torso oscillates and lengthens almost imperceptibly with the breath. Eventually you may be able to stretch the arms out beyond the feet on the floor.

Stay in the pose anywhere from 1 to 3 minutes. To come up, first lift the torso away from the thighs and straighten the elbows again if they are bent. Then inhale and lift the torso up by pulling the tailbone down and into the pelvis.

Bound Angle Pose - Baddha Konasana

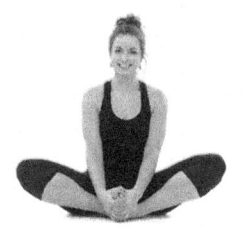

Bound Angle Pose, also called Cobbler's Pose after the typical sitting position of Indian cobblers, is an excellent groin and hip-opener.

YOGA BASICS

Benefits include:

- Stimulates abdominal organs, ovaries and prostate gland, bladder, and kidneys
- Stimulates the heart and improves general circulation
- Stretches the inner thighs, groins, and knees
- Helps relieve mild depression, anxiety, and fatigue
- Soothes menstrual discomfort and sciatica
- Helps relieve the symptoms of menopause
- Therapeutic for flat feet, high blood pressure, infertility, and asthma
- Consistent practice of this pose until late into pregnancy is said to help ease childbirth
- Traditional texts say that Baddha Konasana destroys disease and gets rid of fatigue

Sit with your legs straight out in front of you, raising your pelvis on a blanket if your hips or groins are tight. Exhale, bend your knees, pull your heels toward your pelvis, then drop your knees out to the sides and press the soles of your feet together.

Bring your heels as close to your pelvis as you comfortably can. With the first and second finger and thumb, grasp the big toe of each foot. Always keep the outer edges of the feet firmly on the floor. If it isn't possible to hold the toes, clasp each hand around the same-side ankle or shin.

Sit so that the pubis in front and the tailbone in back are equidistant from the floor. The perineum then will be approximately parallel to the floor and the pelvis in a neutral position. Firm the sacrum and shoulder blades against the back and lengthen the front torso through the top of the sternum.

Never force your knees down. Instead release the heads of the thigh bones toward the floor. When this action leads, the knees follow.

Stay in this pose anywhere from 1 to 5 minutes. Then inhale, lift your knees away from the floor, and extend the legs back to their original position.

Wide-Angle Seated Forward Bend - Upavistha Konasana

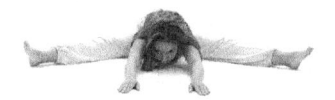

Upavistha Konasana is a good preparation for most of the seated forward bends and twists, as well as the wide-leg standing poses.

Benefits include:

- Stretches the insides and backs of the legs
- Stimulates the abdominal organs
- Strengthens the spine
- Calms the brain
- Releases groins

Use caution with this exercise if you have a lower back injury.

Sit with your legs extended out in front of you, then lean your torso back slightly on your hands and lift and open your legs to an angle of about 90 degrees (the legs should form an approximate right angle, with the pubis at the apex). Press your hands against the floor and slide your buttocks forward, widening the legs another 10 to 20 degrees. If you can't sit comfortably on the floor, raise your buttocks on a folded blanket.

Rotate your thighs outwardly, pinning the outer thighs against the floor, so that the knee caps point straight up toward the ceiling. Reach out through your heels and stretch your soles, pressing though the balls of the feet.

With your thigh bones pressed heavily into the floor and your knee caps pointing up at the ceiling, walk your hands forward between your legs. Keep your arms long.

As with all forward bends, the emphasis is on moving from the hip joints and maintaining the length of the front torso. As soon as you find yourself bending from the waist, stop, re-establish the length from the pubis to the navel, and continue forward if possible.

Increase the forward bend on each exhalation until you feel a comfortable stretch in the backs of your legs. Stay in the pose 1 minute or longer. Then come up on an inhalation with a long front torso.

Full Boat Pose

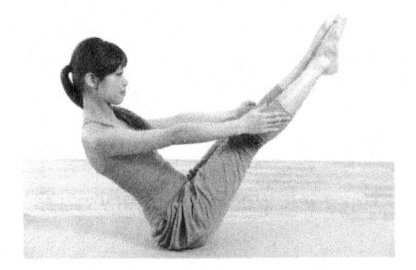

An abdominal and deep hip flexor strengthener, Boat Pose requires you to balance on the tripod of your sitting bones and tailbone.

Benefits include:

- Strengthens the abdomen, hip flexors, and spine

- Stimulates the kidneys, thyroid and prostate glands, and intestines
- Helps relieve stress
- Improves digestion

Use caution if you have low blood pressure, insomnia, neck problems, are pregnant or menstruating.

Sit on the floor with your legs straight in front of you. Press your hands on the floor a little behind your hips, fingers pointing toward the feet, and strengthen the arms. Lift through the top of the sternum and lean back slightly. As you do this make sure your back doesn't round; continue to lengthen the front of your torso between the pubis and top sternum. Sit on the "tripod" of your two sitting bones and tailbone.

Exhale and bend your knees, then lift your feet off the floor, so that the thighs are angled about 45-50 degrees relative to the floor. Lengthen your tailbone into the floor and lift your pubis toward your navel. If possible, slowly straighten your knees, raising the tips of your toes slightly above the level of your eyes. If this isn't possible remain with your knees bent, perhaps lifting the shins parallel to the floor.

Stretch your arms alongside the legs, parallel to each other and the floor. Spread the shoulder blades across your back and reach strongly out through the fingers. If this isn't possible, keep the hands on the floor beside your hips or hold on to the backs of your thighs.

While the lower belly should be firm, it shouldn't get hard and thick. Try to keep the lower belly relatively flat. Press the heads of the thigh bones toward the floor to help anchor the pose and lift the top sternum. Breathe easily. Tip the chin slightly toward the sternum so the base of the skull lifts lightly away from the back of the neck.

At first stay in the pose for 10-20 seconds. Gradually increase the time of your stay to 1 minute. Release the legs with an exhalation and sit upright on an inhalation.

Bridge Pose

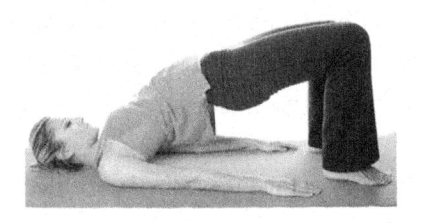

This active version of Bridge Pose calms the brain and rejuvenates tired legs.

Benefits include:

- Stretches the chest, neck, and spine
- Calms the brain and helps alleviate stress and mild depression
- Stimulates abdominal organs, lungs, and thyroid
- Rejuvenates tired legs
- Improves digestion
- Helps relieve the symptoms of menopause
- Relieves menstrual discomfort when done supported
- Reduces anxiety, fatigue, backache, headache, and insomnia
- Therapeutic for asthma, high blood pressure, osteoporosis, and sinusitis

Use caution if you have a neck injury.

Lie supine on the floor, and if necessary, place a thickly folded blanket under your shoulders to protect your neck. Bend your knees and set your feet on the floor, heels as close to the sitting bones as possible.

Exhale and, pressing your inner feet and arms actively into the floor, push your tailbone upward toward the pubis, firming (but not hardening) the buttocks, and lift the buttocks off the floor. Keep your thighs and inner feet parallel. Clasp the hands below your pelvis and extend through the arms to help you stay on the tops of your shoulders.

Lift your buttocks until the thighs are about parallel to the floor. Keep your knees directly over the heels, but push them forward, away from the hips, and lengthen the tailbone toward the backs of the knees. Lift the pubis toward the navel.

Lift your chin slightly away from the sternum and, firming the shoulder blades against your back, press the top of the sternum toward the chin. Firm the outer arms, broaden the shoulder blades, and try to lift the space between them at the base of the neck (where it's resting on the blanket) up into the torso.

Stay in the pose anywhere from 30 seconds to 1 minute. Release with an exhalation, rolling the spine slowly down onto the floor.

Legs-Up-the-Wall Pose - Viparita Karani

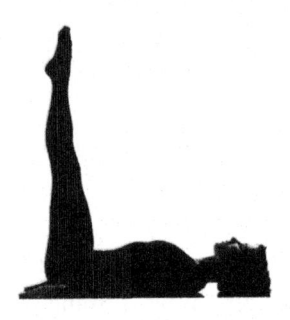

Said to reverse the normal downward flow of a precious subtle fluid called amrita (immortal) or soma (extract) in the Hatha Yoga Pradipika, modern yogis agree that Viparita Karani may have the power to cure whatever ails you.

Benefits include:

- Relieves tired or cramped legs and feet
- Gently stretches the back legs, front torso, and the back of the neck
- Relieves mild backache
- Calms the mind

The pose described this is a passive, supported variation of the shoulder stand. For your support you'll need one or two thickly folded blankets or a firm round bolster. You'll also need to rest your legs vertically (or nearly so) on a wall or other upright support.

Before performing the pose, determine two things about your support: its height and its distance from the wall. If you're stiffer, the support should be lower and placed farther from the wall; if you're more flexible, use a higher support that is closer to the wall.

Your distance from the wall also depends on your height: if you're shorter move closer to the wall, if taller move farther from the wall. Experiment with the position of your support until you find the placement that works for you.

Start with your support about 5 to 6 inches away from the wall. Sit sideways on right end of the support, with your right side against the wall (left-handers can substitute "left" for "right" in these instructions). Exhale and, with one smooth movement, swing your legs up onto the wall and your shoulders and head lightly down onto the floor.

The first few times you do this you may slide off the support and plop down with your buttocks on the floor. Don't get discouraged. Try lowering the support and/or moving it slightly further off the wall until you gain some facility with this movement, then move back closer to the wall.

Your sitting bones don't need to be right against the wall, but they should be "dripping" down into the space between the support and the wall. Check that the front of your torso gently arches from the pubis to the top of the shoulders.

If the front of your torso seems flat, then you've probably slipped a bit off the support. Bend your knees, press your feet into the wall and lift your pelvis off the support a few inches, tuck the support a little higher up under your pelvis, then lower your pelvis onto the support again.

Lift and release the base of your skull away from the back of your neck and soften your throat. Don't push your chin against your sternum; instead let your sternum lift toward the chin. Take a small roll (made from a towel for example) under your neck if the cervical spine feels flat. Open your shoulder blades away from the spine and release your hands and arms out to your sides, palms up.

Keep your legs relatively firm, just enough to hold them vertically in place. Release the heads of the thigh bones and the weight of your belly deeply into your torso, toward the back of the pelvis. Soften your eyes and turn them down to look into your heart.

Stay in this pose anywhere from 5 to 15 minutes. Be sure not to twist off the support when coming out. Instead, slide off the support onto the floor before turning to the side. You can also bend your knees and push your feet against the wall to lift your pelvis off the support. Then slide the support to one side, lower your pelvis to the floor, and turn to the side. Stay on your side for a few breaths, and come up to sitting with an exhalation.

Corpse Pose – Savasana

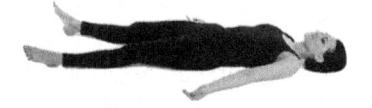

Savasana is a pose of total relaxation—making it one of the most challenging asanas.

Benefits include:

- Calms the brain and helps relieve stress and mild depression
- Relaxes the body
- Reduces headache, fatigue, and insomnia
- Helps to lower blood pressure

In Savasana it's essential that the body be placed in a neutral position. Sit on the floor with your knees bent, feet on the floor, and lean back onto your forearms. Lift your pelvis slightly off the floor and, with your hands, push the back of the pelvis toward the tailbone, then return the pelvis to the floor.

Inhale and slowly extend the right leg, then the left, pushing through the heels. Release both legs, softening the groins, and see that the legs are angled evenly relative to the mid-line of the torso, and that the feet turn out equally. You should narrow the front pelvis and soften (but don't flatten) the lower back.

With your hands lift the base of the skull away from the back of the neck and release the back of the neck down toward the tailbone. If you have any difficulty doing this, support the back of the head and neck on a folded blanket. Broaden the base of the skull too, and lift the crease of the neck diagonally into the center of the head. Make sure your ears are equidistant from your shoulders.

Reach your arms toward the ceiling, perpendicular to the floor. Rock slightly from side to side and broaden the back ribs and the shoulder blades away from the spine. Then release the arms to the floor, angled evenly relative to the mid-line of torso.

Turn the arms outward and stretch them away from the space between the shoulder blades. Rest the backs of the hands on the floor as close as you comfortably can to the index finger knuckles. Make sure the shoulder blades are resting evenly on the floor. Imagine the lower tips of the shoulder blades are lifting diagonally into your back toward the top of the sternum. From here, spread the collarbones.

In addition to quieting the physical body in Savasana, it's also necessary to pacify the sense organs. Soften the root of the tongue, the wings of the nose, the channels of the inner ears, and the skin of the forehead, especially around the bridge of the nose between the eyebrows. Let the eyes sink to the back of the head, then turn them downward to gaze at the heart. Release your brain to the back of the head.

Stay in this pose for 5 minutes for every 30 minutes of practice. To exit, first roll gently with an exhalation onto one side, preferably the right. Take 2 or 3 breaths. With another exhalation press your hands against the floor and lift your torso, dragging your head slowly after. The head should always come up last.

After completing these exercises, take a few moments to practice some deep meditation which is covered in the next section.

Chapter 7: What Is Meditation?

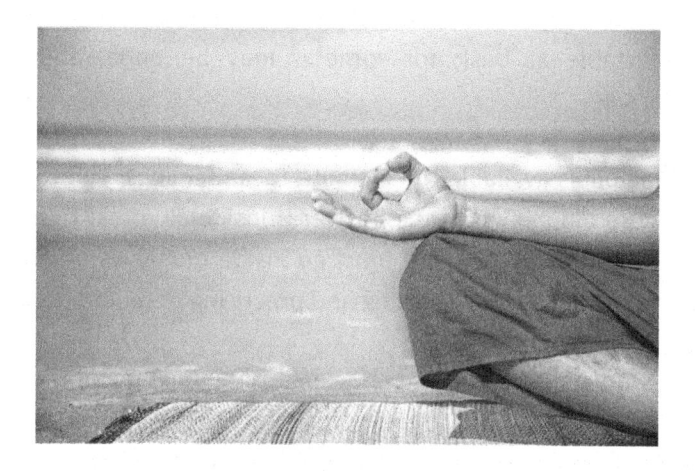

Meditation can be more accurately called relaxation. It is striving to reach a state of serenity within your body and mind. Achieving a balance between the two can lead you to self-actualization and inner peace. Who couldn't use that?

Meditating is actually easier than you might imagine. Most of us have probably dabbled in meditation by participating in conscious relaxation – perhaps during an exercise class or to manage pain at the dentist or anxiety before a test. We start by paying attention to our breathing. The practical effort of meditation is to focus completely on our breathing taking our minds away from the "mind clutter" that constantly tries to invade our mind and eliminates feelings that will lead to a time of calm.

With repeated effort the goal of clearing your mind – to think of nothing, does occur and the process of meditation takes on its own energy. The result is peace, serenity, calmness, eventually opening you to new insights.

Our world can be fast, fun and exciting. It is also challenging, trying, demanding and frightening. These two sides of our lives produce stress, emotional reactions, anxiety, worry and anticipation. Our bodies and minds can tolerate only so much of any of these. After a while, each of us reaches a saturation point and the results become uncomfortable at best; for some it may be unbearable, even unendurable.

No magic pill is available to eliminate these feelings. The reality is, as the wise old man said, the answer is inside all of us. To manage these universal concerns we must go inside ourselves. Among the steps we can take is the learning and practicing of meditation.

There is no right or wrong behavior during your meditation. It is your time for you. Everyone deserves this kind of personal attention. This is a self-care activity; loving oneself!

Teach it to your children instead of a time-out in their room or corner. Teach it to your friends, family, anyone who will listen. We can share this gift and get back as we give. We are all better because of each person who meditates. The peace and joy felt by those who meditate enters the world for all of us as positive energy. From it the world is a better place.

So what exactly is meditation? There are many types of meditation. The one definition that fits almost all types is..."Consciously directing your attention to alter your state of consciousness."

There's no limit to the things you can direct your attention toward...symbols, sounds, colors, breath, uplifting thoughts, spiritual realms, etc. Meditation is simply about attention...where you direct it, and how it alters your consciousness.

Traditionally meditation was (and still is) used for spiritual growth...i.e. becoming more conscious; unfolding our inner Light,

Love, & Wisdom; becoming more aware of the guiding Presence in our lives; accelerating our journey home to our True Self... our Spirit.

More recently, meditation has become a valuable tool for finding a peaceful oasis of relaxation and stress relief in a demanding, fast-paced world.

It can be used for healing, emotional cleansing and balancing, deepening concentration, unlocking creativity, and finding inner guidance. Meditating is also the culmination of yoga exercises as your body reaches a state of relaxation, so should your mind.

When you begin your meditation, put your expectations aside, and don't worry about doing it right. There are infinite possibilities and no fixed criterion for determining right meditation. There are, however, a few things to avoid. Don't try to force something to happen. Don't over-analyze the meditation and don't try to make your mind blank or chase thoughts away. There is no one "right" way to meditate, so just concentrate on the process and find the best way for YOU!

Find a quiet, comfortable place to meditate. You can sit in a comfortable chair, on the bed, on the floor...anywhere that's comfortable. It's not necessary to sit cross-legged. Your legs can be in any position that is comfortable. Eliminate as much noise and as many potential distractions as possible. Don't worry about those things that you cannot control.

When you sit to meditate, sit comfortably, with your spine reasonably straight. This allows the spiritual energy to flow freely up the spine, which is an important aspect of meditation. Leaning against a chair back, a wall, headboard, etc. is perfectly all right. If, for physical reasons, you can't sit up, lay flat on your back. Place your hands in any position that is comfortable.

There are many types of meditation you can practice. We'll explore some of the more popular and effective ones.

UNIVERSAL MANTRA MEDITATION

This meditation comes from an ancient Indian text called the Malini Vijaya Tantra, which dates back about 5000 years. It is a very easy meditation, yet very powerful in its capacity to quiet your mind and connect you with your Essence or Inner Spirit.

This meditation uses a mantra as your object of focus. A mantra is a word or phrase that has the power to catalyze a shift into deeper, more peaceful states of awareness. The mantra most use for this meditation is: Aum. Aum does not have a literal translation. Rather, it is the essential vibration of the universe. If you were to tune into the actual sound of the cosmos, the perpetual sound of Aummm is what you would hear.

Although this mantra is sometimes chanted aloud, in this meditation, you will be repeating the mantra mentally...silently. Before we get to the actual steps, there are a few important points to be aware of.

- One of the keys to this meditation is repeating the mantra gently or faintly in your mind.
- The power of this technique comes from letting go and allowing your attention to dive into the deeper realms of awareness. Therefore, even though you will be focusing on the mantra, staying focused on the mantra is not the aim of this meditation. Trying too hard to stay focused would keep your attention from descending into the deeper realms. Instead, you will be repeating the mantra with "minimal effort", and giving your mind the space to wander a bit.

- Resist the temptation to make something happen, and allow the mantra to do the work.

This meditation easily produces a shift into deeper, more peaceful states of awareness. (The degree of this will vary from session to session.) It increases the flow of energy to the brain and clears away a good deal of physical and emotional toxins.

Because of this detoxification, it is best to keep this meditation to 10 or 15 minutes a day when first beginning. After a month or so, it can be increased to 20 minutes, but that should be the maximum for anyone who does not have quite a few years of meditation experience. Also, it is advisable to drink a lot of pure water. Finally, mantra meditation accelerates spiritual growth as you achieve a state of relaxation and self-awareness.

1. Sit comfortably, with your eyes closed and your spine reasonably straight.
2. Begin repeating the mantra gently in your mind.
3. Repeat the mantra at whatever tempo feels most natural. There is no need to synchronize the mantra with your breathing, but if this occurs naturally, it's ok.
4. Allow the mantra to arise more faintly in your mind...repeating it with minimal effort.
5. Continue repeating the mantra faintly, and allow for whatever happens.
6. If at any time, you feel that you are slipping into a sleep-like or dream-like state, allow it to happen.
7. If and when you notice that your attention has drifted completely off the mantra, gently begin repeating it again, and continue with minimal effort.
8. After 10 or 15 minutes, stop repeating the mantra, and come out of your meditation slowly.

RELAXATION MEDITATION

This remarkably easy and relaxing meditation makes use of a little-known secret about the eyes. Allowing the eyes to rest in a soft downward gaze has an instant, automatic relaxing effect. Relaxation meditation provides a great deal of stress reduction and can be used as a quick 2 minute relax and refresh break almost anywhere. You will also realize a heightened sense of alertness.

1. Sit comfortably with your spine reasonably straight.
2. Allow your eyes to rest comfortably downward, gazing softly, but not focused on anything.
3. Without closing your eyes completely, let your eyelids drop to a level that feels most comfortable.
4. Continue gazing downward...the act of gazing is your primary focus (rather than the area at which you are gazing). You may notice your breathing becoming more rhythmic.
5. It's ok to let your attention drift a bit. If your eyes become very heavy, it's ok to let them close. If you notice you've come out of your relaxed space, simply bring your attention back to your relaxed downward gaze.

ENERGY HEALING MEDITATION

In this simple healing meditation, you send the powerful healing Life Force directly to the area in need of help. This Life Force is the energy behind all healing. Wherever this energy is flowing and in balance, there is health and well-being. Wherever this energy is blocked or out of balance, illness manifests.

Many people believe in visualization as a key healing tool. Energy healing meditation helps you to concentrate your positive energy on an afflicted area and alleviate any adverse symptoms and feelings that are being manifested through the physical pain.

1. Sit reasonably straight and close your eyes.
2. Breathe slowly, as silently as possible. (Holding your breath after inhaling or exhaling is not recommended.)
3. As you inhale, feel yourself breathing the healing Life Force in through your solar plexus. Picture this Life Force as a very refined, light energy.
4. As you exhale, gently direct this light energy to the afflicted area. If there is not a specific ailing area, disperse this light energy throughout your body as you exhale.
5. Continue until you feel the area has received enough Life Force.

COLOR HEALING MEDITATION

We are not just our physical selves. We are multi-dimensional beings, composed of an Inner Spirit, a mental body, an emotional body, a vital body, and a physical body. The energy of these bodies becomes progressively subtler from physical to spiritual. Illness begins with disharmony in one of these energy bodies. If not harmonized, the disease moves outward, affecting the denser bodies, ultimately manifesting as physical illness.

Total healing requires restoring harmony to all of our bodies. This meditation is designed to cleanse and harmonize your various bodies with the healing energies of color.

Color healing meditation will provide you with cleansing, balancing, & healing at all levels: Spiritual, Mental, Emotional, Vital, & Physical. It also will develop concentration & visualization abilities.

1. Sit comfortably with your eyes closed.
2. Visualize a large ball of radiant Golden light a few inches over your head. Visualize that ball of light slowly descending through your crown, filling your entire being with golden light.

3. Imagine yourself absorbing that light as it nourishes, cleanses and heals your whole being - your Spirit and all of your bodies - dissolving all blocked and toxic energies.
4. Repeat this exercise, visualizing a ball of Red light. Continue through the entire spectrum like this, visualizing a ball of Orange light; Yellow light; Green light; Blue light; Indigo light; and Violet light. Go through the spectrum at whatever pace feels appropriate.
5. Take some time to visualize yourself in a state of perfect, radiant health.

CENTERING

Centering is meditation in action. Within you is a space that is always calm and at peace. This space is often referred to as your "calm center". Being centered means remaining in your calm center amidst the busyness of everyday life. Being centered means not allowing your inner light to be overshadowed by stressful circumstances or negative thoughts and emotions.

When you are centered, you are in a state of clarity, focus, peace, and balance. When you are not centered, you are unclear, unfocussed, stressed, and off balance.

A good centering technique will require only minimal attention, allowing you to keep some of your attention on the activity at hand. Here are some very easy, effective centering techniques.

1. **Simple Breath Awareness** - While involved in whatever you are doing, bring some attention to your breathing for just a few moments...it needn't be your full attention...just enough to bring you back to your calm center. Breathe naturally, or perhaps just a little more slowly and deeply.
2. **Reclaiming Your Energy** - When you are feeling stressed and scattered, take several slow, deep breaths. With each

in-breath, imagine you are pulling all of your scattered energy and attention back to your inner self...your calm center.

Letting Go - This centering technique combines breath awareness with the phrase or mantra, "Let go." It is especially helpful when you are tense and/or fixating on a stressful situation or a negative thought or emotion. As you inhale, (silently or aloud) say, "Let" as you exhale, say "go"...while letting go of all that is stressing you.

Inner Sun - Imagine a bright sun filling your heart chakra...the calm, subtle energy field that permeates your chest area. Imagine that sun gently emanating peace and joy throughout your entire being.

Yoga and meditation certainly have proven to be effective tools to lessen stress and provide a sense of calm that cannot be achieved through conventional exercise. So what about those stress-filled days at the office when you are unable to concentrate on work because of outside distractions? You can perform yoga right at your desk if you want! Let's look at "desktop yoga".

Chapter 8: Yoga at Your Desk

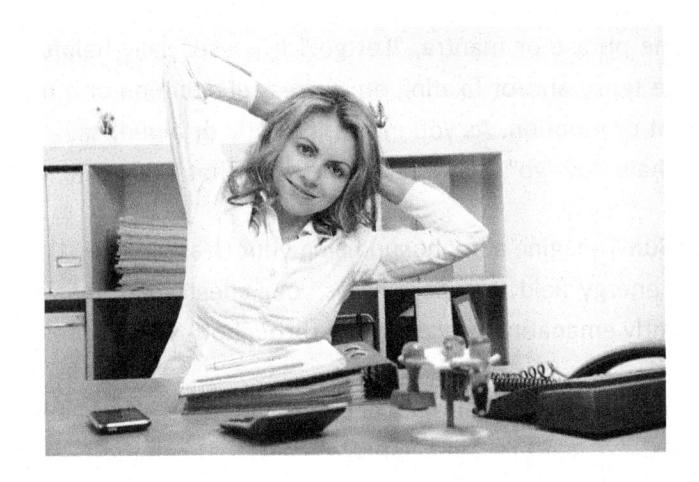

Whether you're a high-powered executive or an administrative assistant with your boss's problems becoming your own, many people in the business world experience an inordinate amount of stress at the office. It would be nice to have a quiet place to practice conventional yoga techniques, but that isn't always possible.

Yoga experts have devised a way for you to do a short yoga program right at your desk. Try these exercises to de-stress at the office.

- Sit up tall in your chair, or if possible stand up. Stretch your arms overhead and interlock your fingers, turn the palms to the ceiling. Take a deep breath in and on the exhale extend your side torso and take the tips of the shoulder blades into the body. Take another deep breath and on the exhale stretch to the right, inhale come up and exhale stretch to the left.

- On an inhale, lift your shoulders up to your ears and then exhale and let them drop. Repeat 3 times. Contract the shoulder muscle fully when you lift your shoulders up and then on the drop it will release more completely.
- Stand (or sit at your desk) with your feet planted firmly in the ground. Inhale and raise the arms out to the side, palms down. Exhale and rotate the palms up, rolling the shoulders back. Take an inhale and on the exhale, bend the elbows in toward the waist. Inhale and on the exhale bring the palms to the belly. This exercise helps to open the chest and extend the upper back.
- Take your hands behind your back and interlock the fingers, stretching the shoulders back, opening the chest. Take several breaths. Make sure that your head stays in the mid-line and that your eye gaze is on the horizon.
- Stand by the wall, extend your right arm and place the palm on the wall with the fingers up. On an exhale, turn your chest away, taking the shoulder blade into the torso.
- Stand by your desk and place your palms on the desk top with the fingers pointing toward your body. Gently stretch the lower arm and wrist.
- Wrap the right arm around the torso and place your right hand on the left shoulder with the elbow at chest height and facing forward. Put your left hand on the right elbow and on an exhale, stretch it toward the left, opening between the shoulder blades. Hold for several breaths and then release. Repeat on the other side.
- Reach the right arm into the air and on an exhale bend the elbow and reach your fingers down the back, between the shoulder blades. Place the left hand on the elbow and on an exhale gently pull the elbow to the left. Relax the ribs and hold for several breaths. Release and repeat on the other side.
- Hug your arms around your chest and then put one elbow underneath the other, the hand facing toward each other and

fingers to the ceiling. Exhale and slowly raise the arms so that the elbows come up to the height of the shoulder, keep the shoulders down. Repeat on the other side.
- Sit on your chair and pull back away from the desk, resting your palms on the desk top and extend your side torso. Lift the ribs up, let the shoulder blades slide towards the desk, and make sure the head is extended from the spine with the chin towards the chest.
- Sit on your chair, feet planted firmly in the floor, sitting bones pressing into the chair. Extend the side torso, and twist to the right (on an exhale), one hand on back to chair, one hand on the side of the chair. Hold for a few breaths and then repeat the other side.
- Sit forward on your chair and open the legs a little wider than the hips. Lean forward from the hips and drop your torso down. Let the head and arms hang down toward the floor.
- Sit upright in your chair with your feet planted firmly on the ground. Press your sitting bones down into the chair and extend the side torso. Relax your shoulders. Place your palms on your knees and spread the fingers wide. Take a deep breath in and on the exhale extend your tongue to your chin; focus your eyes to your nose. Inhale and bring the tongue back into the mouth. Exhale and stick the tongue out again and this time focus the eyes up to your forehead. Repeat 3 times.
- Sit upright on chair, relax your shoulders and extend the side torso up. Relax your facial muscles, the jaw and tongue. Circle the eyes clockwise 8 times and counter-clockwise 8 times. Close your eyes and breathe deeply for a few slow breaths.

Yoga can be used for more than simple de-stressing. It can also be used to alleviate the symptoms of everyday ailments without the use of medication.

Chapter 9: Yoga Poses to Relieve Headaches, Cramps and Depression

YOGA FOR HEADACHES

There are many different kinds of headaches. Some (like tension headaches, sinus headaches and migraines) are fairly common; others (like headaches caused by brain tumors) are relatively rare. Various treatments are recommended for dealing with headaches. Yoga asanas and breathing can help too, though mostly with tension-type headaches.

Everyone gets a tension headache now and again, but if you suffer from this type of headache habitually, it's important to consult a doctor or other health practitioner to treat the pain and work to resolve the ultimate source of the tension.

When treating a tension headache with asanas and breathing, it's important to start practicing as soon as possible after you start to feel the pain. Once the headache is established it will be very difficult to alleviate.

Here are the yoga positions that can be used to alleviate a headache:

Child's Pose (Balasana)

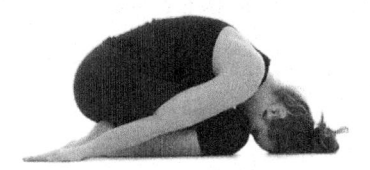

1. Kneel on the floor. Touch your big toes together and sit on your heels, then separate your knees about as wide as your hips.
2. Exhale and lay your torso down between your thighs. Broaden your sacrum across the back of your pelvis and narrow your hip points toward the navel, so that they nestle down onto the inner thighs. Lengthen your tailbone away from the back of the pelvis while you lift the base of your skull away from the back of your neck.
3. Lay your hands on the floor alongside your torso, palms up, and release the fronts of your shoulders toward the floor. Feel how the weight of the front shoulders pulls the shoulder blades wide across your back.
4. Balasana is a resting pose. Stay anywhere from 30 seconds to a few minutes. Beginners can also use Balasana to get a taste of a deep forward bend, where the torso rests on the thighs. Stay in the pose from 1 to 3 minutes. To come up, first lengthen the front torso, and then with an inhalation lift from the tailbone as it presses down and into the pelvis.

Note: you can do the child's pose when you get tired, out of breath, or need to rest. Simply pick up with your exercises again when refreshed. Child's pose is also a great way to quickly alleviate stress at any time.

Standing Forward Bend

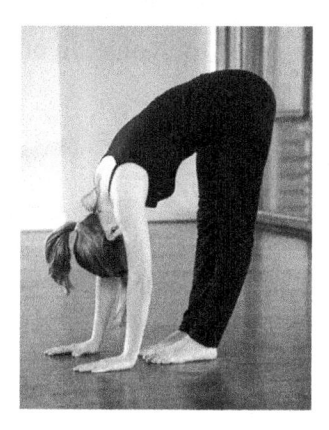

1. Stand in relaxed position with your hands on your hips. Exhale and bend forward from the hip joints, not from the waist. As you descend draw the front torso out of the groins and open the space between the pubis and top sternum. As in all the forward bends, the emphasis is on lengthening the front torso as you move more fully into the position.
2. If possible, with your knees straight, bring your palms or finger tips to the floor slightly in front of or beside your feet, or bring your palms to the backs of your ankles. If this isn't possible, cross your forearms and hold your elbows. Press the heels firmly into the floor and lift the sitting bones toward the ceiling. Turn the top thighs slightly inward.
3. With each inhalation in the pose, lift and lengthen the front torso just slightly; with each exhalation release a little more fully into the forward bend. In this way the torso oscillates almost imperceptibly with the breath. Let your head hang from the root of the neck, which is deep in the upper back, between the shoulder blades.
4. This pose can be used as a resting position between the standing poses. Stay in the pose for 30 seconds to 1 minute. It can also be practiced as a pose in itself.

5. Don't roll the spine to come up. Instead bring your hands back onto your hips and reaffirm the length of the front torso. Then press your tailbone down and into the pelvis and come up on an inhalation with a long front torso.

Bridge Pose

Corpse Pose

Downward Facing Dog

Legs Up The Wall

Standing Forward Bend

YOGA FOR MENSTRUAL CRAMPS

Menstrual cramps can be very debilitating for those who suffer from severe cramps early in their cycle. While your first inclination might be to lie on your couch in the fetus position moaning in pain, try yoga to relieve the pain.

Exercise during menstruation is generally highly recommended. It's believed that exercise can ease the discomfort of your period; quell mood swings, anxiety, and depression; and reduce bloating.

Most contemporary yoga teachers advise a fairly conservative approach toward asana practice during menstruation. This makes perfect sense for women who feel sluggish during their cycle.

However, many other women don't feel the need to change anything about their practice during menstruation, except maybe to limit strenuous inverted poses. Each student should decide for herself what kind of asana sequence is most appropriate for her body during menstruation.

Reclining Bound Angle

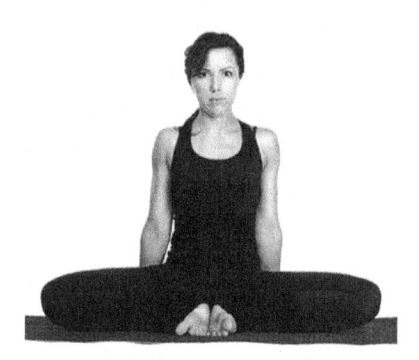

1. Sit with the soles of your feet touching each other. Exhale and lower your back torso toward the floor, first leaning on your hands.
2. Once you are leaning back on your forearms, use your hands to spread the back of your pelvis and release your lower back and upper buttocks through your tailbone. Bring your torso all the way to the floor, supporting your head and neck on a blanket roll or bolster if needed.
3. With your hands grip your topmost thighs and rotate your inner thighs externally, pressing your outer thighs away from the sides of your torso. Next slide your hands along your outer thighs from the hips toward the knees and widen your outer knees away from your hips.
4. Then slide your hands down along your inner thighs, from the knees to the groins. Imagine that your inner groins are sinking into your pelvis. Push your hip points together, so that while the back pelvis widens, the front pelvis narrows. Lay your arms on the floor, angled at about 45 degrees from the sides of your torso, palms up.

The natural tendency in this pose is to push the knees toward the floor in the belief that this will increase the stretch of the inner thighs and groins. But especially if your groins are tight, pushing the knees down will have just the opposite of the intended effect: The groins will harden, as

- will your belly and lower back. Instead, imagine that your knees are floating up toward the ceiling and continue settling your groins deep into your pelvis. As your groins drop toward the floor, so will your knees.
- To start, stay in this pose for one minute. Gradually extend your stay anywhere from five to 10 minutes. To come out, use your hands to press your thighs together, then roll over onto one side and push yourself away from the floor, head trailing the torso.
- Move back into sitting position with the soles of your feet touching.

Upward Bow

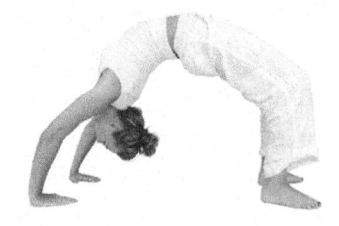

Basically, this is a simple back bend. Lay on the floor, place your hands above your head flat on the floor and raise your back into an arched position.

Seated Twist

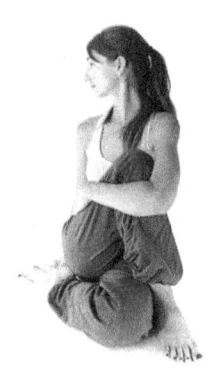

Still sitting twist to the right with an exhalation, hold for 30 seconds, then twist to the left for 30 seconds. Repeat three times to each side, each time holding for 30 seconds.

Corpse Pose

Legs Up the Wall

Seated Forward Bend

Wide Angle Seated Forward Bend

YOGA FOR DEPRESSION

The word "depression" covers a wide range of conditions, from long-standing and severe clinical or major depression to shorter-term and episodic mild depression, to situational depression brought on by a major life change, such as the death of a spouse, job loss, divorce.

Many different therapies are available for depression, including anti-depressants and psychotherapy. Studies indicate that regular exercise too, including yoga asanas and breathing, can help some people ease the symptoms of mild to moderate forms of depression.

Of course, one major hurdle in using exercise to alleviate depression is motivation, or lack of it. Most depressed people don't really feel much like getting out of bed in the morning, much less exercising.

Then too, failure to see the exercise program through can make a depressed person feel even worse. So start off slowly, and be sure to choose an exercise that you really enjoy; if possible, exercise with a supportive partner or group. Try to exercise at least three times a week.

Headstand

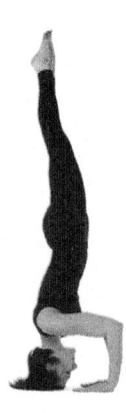

1. Use a folded blanket or sticky mat to pad your head and forearms. Kneel on the floor. Lace your fingers together and set the forearms on the floor, elbows at shoulder width.
2. Roll the upper arms slightly outward, but press the inner wrists firmly into the floor. Set the crown of your head on the floor.
3. If you are just beginning to practice this pose, press the bases of your palms together and snuggle the back of your head against the clasped hands. More experienced students can

open their hands and place the back of the head into the open palms.
4. Inhale and lift your knees off the floor. Carefully walk your feet closer to your elbows, heels elevated. Actively lift through the top thighs, forming an inverted "V."
5. Firm the shoulder blades against your back and lift them toward the tailbone so the front torso stays as long as possible. This should help prevent the weight of the shoulders collapsing onto your neck and head.
6. Exhale and lift your feet away from the floor. Take both feet up at the same time, even if it means bending your knees and hopping lightly off the floor. As the legs (or thighs, if your knees are bent) rise to perpendicular to the floor, firm the tailbone against the back of the pelvis.
7. Turn the upper thighs in slightly, and actively press the heels toward the ceiling (straightening the knees if you bent them to come up). The center of the arches should align over the center of the pelvis, which in turn should align over the crown of the head.
8. Firm the outer arms inward, and soften the fingers. Continue to press the shoulder blades against the back, widen them, and draw them toward the tailbone. Keep the weight evenly balanced on the two forearms.
9. It's also essential that your tailbone continues to lift upward toward the heels. Once the backs of the legs are fully lengthened through the heels, maintain that length and press up through the balls of the big toes so the inner legs are slightly longer than the outer.
10. As a beginner, stay in this position for 10 seconds. Gradually add 5 to 10 seconds onto your stay every day or so until you can comfortably hold the pose for 3 minutes. Then continue for 3 minutes each day for a week or two, until you feel relatively comfortable in the pose.

11. Again gradually add 5 to 10 seconds onto your stay every day or so until you can comfortably hold the pose for 5 minutes. Come down with an exhalation, without losing the lift of the shoulder blades, with both feet touching the floor at the same time.

Head to Knee Forward Bend

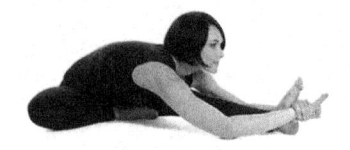

Benefits Include:

- Calms the brain and helps relieve mild depression
- Stretches the spine, shoulders, hamstrings, and groin
- Stimulates the liver and kidneys
- Improves digestion
- Helps relieve the symptoms of menopause
- Relieves anxiety, fatigue, headache, menstrual discomfort
- Therapeutic for high blood pressure, insomnia, and sinusitis
- Strengthens the back muscles during pregnancy (up to second trimester), done without coming forward, keeping your back spine concave and front torso long.

Use caution with this pose if you have a knee injury.

1. Sit on the floor with your buttocks lifted on a folded blanket and your legs straight in front of you. Inhale, bend your right knee, and draw the heel back toward your perineum. Rest your right foot sole lightly against your inner left thigh, and lay the

outer right leg on the floor, with the shin at a right angle to the left leg (if your right knee doesn't rest comfortably on the floor, support it with a folded blanket).
2. Press your right hand against the inner right groin, where the thigh joins the pelvis, and your left hand on the floor beside the hip. Exhale and turn the torso slightly to the left, lifting the torso as you push down on and ground the inner right thigh. Line up your navel with the middle of the left thigh. You can just stay here, using a strap to help you lengthen the spine evenly, grounding through the sitting bones.
3. Or, when you are ready, you can drop the strap and reach out with your right hand to take the inner left foot, thumb on the sole. Inhale and lift the front torso, pressing the top of the left thigh into the floor and extending actively through the left heel. Use the pressure of the left hand on the floor to increase the twist to the left. Then reach your left hand to the outside of the foot. With the arms fully extended, lengthen the front torso from the pubis to the top of the sternum.
4. Exhale and extend forward from the groins, not the hips. Be sure not to pull yourself forcefully into the forward bend, hunching the back and shortening the front torso. As you descend, bend your elbows out to the sides and lift them away from the floor.
5. Lengthen forward into a comfortable stretch. The lower belly should touch the thighs first, the head last. Stay in the pose anywhere from 1 to 3 minutes. Come up with an inhalation and repeat the instructions with the legs reversed for the same length of time.

Bridge Pose

Corpse Pose

Downward Facing Dog

Reclining Bound Angle

Seated Twist

Standing Forward Bend

Legs Up The Wall

Upward Bow

Chapter 10: Conclusion

The popularity of yoga is, without a doubt, increasing as people are constantly trying to balance the stresses of everyday life with their own spiritual well-being.

It is important for you, the reader, to realize that we are not medical professionals and have simply tried to provide you with an introduction to yoga and meditation. This book is a way for you to get started on your own yoga program.

If you have special health considerations, you should be sure and consult with your doctor before embarking on a yoga program, or any other exercise program for that matter. We cannot be held responsible in any way for any problems that may arise from your yoga journey. This is meant simply as an informational tool to help you start down that path.

But you will find that once you start initiating yoga into your daily exercise routine, you will most likely notice a heightened state of well-being and a more spiritual connection to both your inner self as well as any higher power you choose to acknowledge.

Remember to concentrate on your breathing when performing the poses, and don't force your body into positions it isn't comfortable doing. When meditating, focus on the inner calm you are trying to achieve.

Perform these exercises when you get the chance. You don't have to do a full cycle to feel better. Even practicing one exercise when you have the time can have huge therapeutic benefits to mind, body, and soul!

Yoga can better your life in so many ways. It can help you become a better spouse, parent, worker, and person. You can help others by spreading your experiences with yoga and meditation. Imagine the thanks you'll receive as you tell others how this ancient art has enhanced your life!

Shanti (peace) to you as you journey to your own Shambhala (place of utter tranquility).

MEET THE AUTHOR

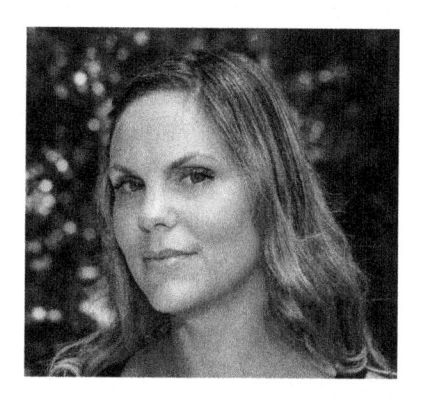

Kim Fyffe leads her clients toward peace and wellness. Sometimes that means perfecting Downward Dog, and sometimes it means addressing medical complexities through nutrition and stress management. Kim has years of experience in the areas of holistic health, yoga, and meditation. She uses her experience in these areas to help people find drive, clarity, and focus.

Though Kim began practicing yoga as a teenager, she really took it to the next level in her early thirties. Mom to two very rambunctious twin boys, she had to admit that she was overwhelmed and overstimulated by 6 o'clock each night. On their third birthday, her husband gave her a gift—a daily yoga pass at the local studio. He offered to flex his schedule so that she could take the time to re-center regularly. In 2010, she journeyed to the Himalayas with two of her instructors to be trained by some very talented yogis. She came away with a new appreciation for holistic medicine and even the power of deep breathing and meditation in fighting chronic illness.

Over the past four years, Kim has been teaching yoga at a local studio and pursuing various certificates in nutrition and natural healing. Her book, Yoga Basics has been a great help to women just like her who sometimes feel overwhelmed in even the best of circumstances.

Kim and her husband Ben love to travel to new places as often as they can. Although when the boys get to pick, superheroes are usually a theme in their travel.